Greece & Rom

NEW SURVEYS IN THE CLASSICS No. 16

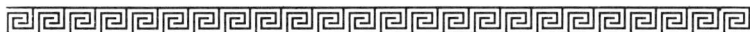

SOPHOCLES

BY

R. G. A. BUXTON

Published for the Classical Association

OXFORD: AT THE CLARENDON PRESS

1984

Oxford University Press, Walton Street, Oxford OX2 6DP

London New York Toronto
Delhi Bombay Calcutta Madras Karachi
Kuala Lumpur Singapore Hong Kong Tokyo
Nairobi Dar es Salaam Cape Town
Melbourne Auckland

and associated companies in
Beirut Berlin Ibadan Mexico City Nicosia

ISBN 0 903035 138

Printed in Great Britain
at the University Press, Oxford
by David Stanford
Printer to the University

PREFACE

This booklet is intended primarily for students at school and university, though I hope it may also be helpful to schoolteachers and to scholars whose expertise lies elsewhere than in Sophoclean studies. In accordance with the general policy of the New Surveys series I have weighted the bibliography in favour of scholarship in English, but I have not hesitated to cite works in other languages where appropriate; nevertheless, in giving references I have usually preferred the shower to the downpour. If what I have written has a bias it is towards literary and dramatic criticism: my aim has been to suggest, in however brief a compass, what Sophocles' plays mean, and where his greatness may be found.

My thanks are due to John Gould and Simon Tremewan for their comments on an earlier draft, and to David Hughes for his generous help with bibliographical matters.

R.G.A.B.

CONTENTS

ABBREVIATIONS

Plays are referred to as follows:

Ant.	*Antigone*
Elec.	*Electra*
Oed. Col.	*Oedipus at Colonus*
Oed. Tyr.	*Oedipus Tyrannus*
Phil.	*Philoctetes*
Trach.	*Trachiniae*

(*Ajax* is not abbreviated)
Periodicals are normally abbreviated as in *L'Année philologique*.

NOTE ON BOOKS AND ARTICLES CITED

Works mentioned once only are cited in full at that point and do not occur in the bibliography. Works mentioned more than once are cited, after the first occurrence, by author's name and date only; such works are listed in the bibliography.

I. RECENT SCHOLARSHIP: SOME POINTERS

So many thousands of scholars have written so many millions of words on Sophocles that one might be forgiven for concluding that there is little prospect of anything valuably new being said. But in fact during the last thirty years our appreciation of this dramatist has been considerably deepened and enriched.[1] It is not that there has been (as with, say, Menander) a great increase in the quantity of material available: nothing of comparable length has turned up since the fragmentary *Ichneutae* discovered near the beginning of this century,[2] so that as ever we must fall back on the seven fully extant tragedies. Yet, as will be evident from the chapters which follow, scholars have been engaged in a genuinely fruitful debate about the issues at stake in the plays.

This debate has been remarkable for the variety of often conflicting critical approaches which participants in it have deployed. One line of enquiry has concentrated on the complex language found in Sophocles, showing how it may contribute to the overall meaning; by contrast other critics have stressed the importance of stage action as a vehicle for meaning (see ch. III). Another focus of debate has been 'character', a problematic notion whose analysis has called into question long-cherished assumptions about the straightforwardness of 'psychological' readings of the behaviour of stage-figures (see ch. IV). A third area of controversy has centred on the supposed piety of Sophocles: are we to see him as advocating humble submission by mortals to the purposes of the gods, or as applauding the glorious defiance of the noble hero, or is his presentation of the relation between human and divine behaviour a more subtle and ambiguous matter? (see ch. V). It is hardly necessary to add that countless other issues too have been subjected to detailed academic scrutiny (see chs. VI and VII).

It may be the seeming homogeneity of Sophocles' output when compared with that of Aeschylus and Euripides which has led to the large number of general books about him, above all (curiously) in English; and the flow shows no sign of abating.[3] New commentaries have also appeared, though less frequently. Jebb has not been superseded, and remains an indispensable guide;[4] Kamerbeek provides a helpful supplement,[5] and there are good commentaries by Stanford and Easterling on *Ajax* and *Trach.* respectively.[6] The most authoritative texts must now be those produced by R. D. Dawe for Teubner (see ch. II(d)).[7] English-speaking readers have a serviceable translation in the Chicago Complete Greek Tragedies series.[8]

NOTES

1. Anyone wishing to examine Sophoclean studies over the past few decades should begin with H. F. Johansen, 'Sophocles 1939–1959', *Lustrum* 7 (1962), 94–288. Evaluation of more recent scholarship can be found in *Anzeiger für die Altertumswissenschaft* thanks to A. Lesky (20 (1967), 193–216) and H. Strohm (24 (1971), 129–62; 26 (1973), 1–5; 30 (1977), 129–44).

2. We do, though, have a stupendously thorough edition of the fragments by S. Radt, *Tragicorum Graecorum Fragmenta* vol. 4, *Sophocles* (Göttingen, 1977). Still to be consulted is the three-volume commentary on *The Fragments of Sophocles* by A. C. Pearson (Cambridge, 1917). A meticulous papyrological account can be found in R. Carden, *The Papyrus Fragments of Sophocles* (Berlin, 1974).

3. E.g. recently R. P. Winnington-Ingram, *Sophocles: an Interpretation* (Cambridge, 1980); Charles Segal, *Tragedy and Civilization: an Interpretation of Sophocles* (Harvard, 1981); A. Machin, *Cohérence et continuité dans le théâtre de Sophocle* (Haute-Ville, 1981). German scholars have been regrettably reticent about expressing themselves at book-length about Sophocles, being perhaps overawed by the example of Reinhardt.

4. Sir R. C. Jebb (Cambridge, 1883–96).

5. J. C. Kamerbeek, *The Plays of Sophocles* (Leiden, 1953–). This series has now covered all the plays except *Oed. Col.*

6. *Ajax*, ed. W. B. Stanford (London, 1963); *Trach.*, ed. P. E. Easterling (Cambridge, 1982). Other commentaries which may be mentioned are those by G. Kaibel on *Elec.* (Leipzig, 1896, repr. Stuttgart, 1967) and G. Müller on *Ant.* (Heidelberg, 1967) – see the review of this by B. M. W. Knox in *Word and Action* (Baltimore, 1979) 165–82. There are smaller commentaries in English: *Elec.*, by J. H. Kells (Cambridge, 1973); *Oed. Tyr.*, by R. D. Dawe (Cambridge, 1982); *Phil.*, by T. B. L. Webster (Cambridge, 1970).

7. Vol. I: *Ajax, Elec., Oed. Tyr.* (Leipzig, 1975); vol. II: *Trach., Ant., Phil., Oed. Col.* (Leipzig, 1979).

8. Ed. D. Grene and R. Lattimore (Chicago, 1954–7). One may also mention the translation (with commentary) on *Oed. Tyr.* by T. Gould (Prentice-Hall Greek Drama Series, Englewood Cliffs, 1970), the individual version of *Trach.* by Ezra Pound (orig. publ. in *The Hudson Review* 6 (1953–4); Faber edn, London, 1969), and translations of *Oed. Tyr.* by D. Fitts and R. Fitzgerald (London, 1951) and of *Oed. Col.* by R. Fitzgerald (London, 1957).

II. 'FACTS': LIFE, WORKS, MANUSCRIPTS

(n.b. *Test* indicates the section on *Testimonia* in Radt (1977); DID indicates the *didascaliae* in *Tragicorum Graecorum Fragmenta*, vol. 1, ed. B. Snell (Göttingen, 1971).)

(a) *Some dates*

?497/6 or 495/4	Birth.[1] (Other dates, earlier and later, are given, but these two each have some support, from *Marm. Par.* and the *Life* of Sophocles respectively.)
468	Victory in first competition. (*Marm. Par.* (= Jacoby 239) A 56; Plu.*Cim.*8.7; in general, *Test* Hc.) With *Triptolemus*? (Cf. Plin. *N.H.* 18.65 = F 600 Radt.)
443/2	Holds office as Hellenotamias (*IG* I² 202.36 = *Test* 18).
?442	*Antigone*?[2]
441/0	General in campaign against Samos.[3]
438	Victory against Euripides, who was 2nd with a tetralogy including *Alcestis* (hypoth. *Alc.* = DID C 11).
431	Came 2nd; Eurip. was 3rd with (*inter al.*) *Medea* (DID C 12).
420/19	Receives the god Asclepius into his home (*Test* M).[4] (See sect. (c) below.)
?413	? Proboulos at Athens (Aristot. *Rhet.* 1419a25 = *Test* 27).[5]
409	Victory with *Phil.* (hypoth. *Phil.*).
406/5	Death.[1] (Evidence includes hypoth. II to *Oed. Col.*, and *Marm. Par.* (= Jacoby 239, A 64.)
402/1	*Oed. Col.* put on by S.'s grandson, also called Sophocles (hypoth. II to *Oed. Col.*).

(b) *Details of artistic career*

Number of plays written: '123, or, according to others, many more' (*Suda* = *Test* 2); '130, of which 17 are spurious' (Aristophanes of Byzantium, reported in *Life* (*Test* 1.18). A simple – probably too simple – expedient is to emend '17' to '7' and so make the figures correspond.

Number of victories: '20; he was second many times, and never third' (Karystios, reported in *Life* (*Test* 1.8); '24' (*Suda* = *Test* 2); '18' (Diod. Sic. 13. 103.4 = *Test* 85; *IG* II² 2325 = DID A 3a 15). To reconcile these figures the Lenaea has been invoked: 18 victories were (it is argued) at the Dionysia, the rest at the lesser festival.[6]

(c) *How much do we really know?*

Any attempt to construct a biography for Sophocles must rest on (i) the *Life*, preserved in a number of medieval manuscripts; (ii) a wide range of snippets, of which a few are inscriptions, the rest anecdotes or other brief allusions by ancient authors. (All the evidence is gathered at the beginning of Radt (1977).) That we should be extremely cautious in believing such anecdotes told about ancient poets is clear from the way the stories tend to reproduce patterns and stock types of event.[7] Often inventions seem to be based on inferences from literature to life. Thus when we hear of the dispute between the aged Sophocles and his son Iophon (*Test* O) – resolved when Sophocles read from *Oed. Col.* and so dispelled the suggestion that he was senile – we may suspect that the mighty quarrel between Oedipus and Polynices in that play stimulated someone's penchant for biography.[8] When we hear (*Test* 1.3) that, after the victory at Salamis, Sophocles led the singing of the paean, we must reckon with the possibility that this is a fiction designed to show that already in his youth the future poet was marked out for greatness. And when we learn that one version of Sophocles' death (*Test* 1.14; P) had him choke over a grape sent to him by an actor, we cannot fail to notice both the neat irony (n.b. the double link with Dionysus) and the non-tragic absurdity of the occurrence (cf. Aeschylus, said to have been brained by a falling tortoise); as if, through the story-pattern, a more-than-usually august life is balanced by a more-than-usually foolish (but still remarkable) death.

The only aspect of the 'known' facts of Sophocles' life which can with any plausibility be brought to bear on the plays is his alleged 'piety'. The *Life* tells us that he was θεοφιλὴς ... ὡς οὐκ ἄλλος, 'exceptionally loved by the gods' (12); that he was specially favoured by Heracles (ibid.); and that he held the priesthood of Halon (11).[9] Other sources (*Test* M) assert that Sophocles welcomed Asclepius' cult into Athens and was worshipped as 'Dexion'.[10] Starved of biographical data, yet at the same time obliged to confront Sophocles' complex presentation of the relations between gods and men, scholars have made much of these anecdotes. For instance: 'It is a precious detail to find the idol of the Athenians, then a genial, serene, dignified graybeard, conversant with, but untroubled by, the moral and religious contradictions of his great age, doling out eggs to a sacred snake ...'[11] Wilamowitz and Dodds both doubted whether Aeschylus or Euripides would have entertained the new cult-divinity; Dodds explictly linked the pious act with Sophocles' poetry.[12] On the contrast with Aeschylus and Euripides it is surely better to agree with Edelstein that 'if such a man as Sophocles favoured Asclepius, the god must have been a true representative of the divine',[13] i.e. Sophocles was not being over-credulous. But here too we find an implicit confidence that we know what 'such a man as Sophocles' was really like – 'pious'. It is fatal to approach the plays on this basis; we would do well to forget the genial graybeard and remember that Sophocles was young before he was old. If what we expect in the plays is simple piety, we shall miss the complexity and ambiguity which are actually there.[14]

If Sophocles' life is impossible to reconstruct with any probability, his artistic career is not much easier to chart. We have no dates for *Ajax, Elec., Oed. Tyr.,* or *Trach.* The vast majority of books on Sophocles treat *Ajax* as either probably or certainly the earliest surviving work,[15] but the stylistic criteria on which such datings are based have been shown up as very flimsy by the Aeschylean '*Suppliants* papyrus':[16] it is best to follow Jebb[17] and say that some of the apparently Aeschylean features of *Ajax* are 'entirely consonant with the hypothesis of a relatively early date' while by no means entailing such a date. Stylistic chronology at its best can be found in Reinhardt's justly celebrated book,[18] which posits a development from pathos-filled 'monologue'-type plays, characterized by an absence of 'dynamism', towards a form in which the meaning is carried by a freer and more shifting use of dialogue. Full though it is of sensitivity and insight, this work is marred by an excessively linear conception of Sophocles' development.[19] Supposed allusions to historical events have been invoked to bolster the arguments from style, but the results have on the whole been unpersuasive. Knox's virtuoso attempt to fix *Oed. Tyr.* in 425 (by analysing how Sophocles describes the plague) deserves respect but is hardly conclusive;[20] while *Ajax, Elec.,* and *Trach.* have regularly evaded the historian's net.[21]

(d) *Manuscripts*

Ignorant though we are about many features of the transmission of Sophocles' text, we can at least isolate what seem to be the major factors in its survival.[22] Of primary importance was the dramatist's popularity: in his own lifetime his victories – 'one' victory at the Dionysia being, of course, a victory with *four* plays – constitute a startlingly high proportion of his total output; and in the century that followed his place in public favour evidently remained secure. (Demosthenes tells us that Aeschines 'often' played Creon in revivals of *Antigone*.)[23] This popularity was officially codified when, thanks to the fourth-century B.C. politician Lycurgus, authorized texts of Sophocles (and Aeschylus and Euripides) were established.[24] The history of the text between the time of Lycurgus and the first printed edition (1502) is dominated by two centres of scholarship, Alexandria and Byzantium.[25] What survived to reach the hands of Byzantine scholars was the selection of seven plays which we have today, incorporating marginal notes going back to the Alexandrians.[26] The nature of the work done by the Byzantines lies at the root of a continuing controversy over our assessment of the extant manuscripts. Universally agreed to be the best of our two-hundred-or-so witnesses is Laurentianus 32.9 (in Florence; mid to late 10th century); but Parisinus gr. 2712 was, it used to be thought, our next most valuable authority. In 1952 Prof. A. Turyn published a book in which he attempted to undermine the worth of the Parisinus by exposing it as a text edited at Byzantium rather than a possible independent witness.[27] Turyn's view has in turn been contested by R. D. Dawe, who argues that manuscripts rejected by Turyn can indeed provide access to authentic readings, and has sought to show 'how confusingly the various manuscripts can shift their affiliations, and how valuable old readings can filter down to us in only one or two manuscripts'.[28] The situation seemed so fluid to Prof. Kamerbeek that he published his commentaries without an accompanying text.[29] Fortunately the dilemma is less acute for ordinary readers than for editors and commentators: however the textual dispute goes, it is improbable that there will be grave repercussions for the overall interpretation and evaluation of Sophocles.

NOTES

1. For dates of birth and death see F. Jacoby *FGrHist*, on 244 (Apollodoros) F 35; also *Test* B.

2. From hypothesis I to *Ant.* (cf. *Test* 25) we learn that Sophocles' success with the play won him the generalship in the Samian campaign. Is this credible? L. Woodbury, 'Sophocles among the Generals', *Phoenix* 24 (1970), 209–24, thinks it is; K. Reinhardt, *Sophocles* (Eng. tr. Oxford, 1979), p. 240, was dubious. Not incompatible with a date of 442 for *Ant.* is the information that *Ant.* came 32nd in S.'s output (hypoth. I and II to *Ant.* = *Test* 159a–b). As Flickinger showed (*CPh* 5 (1910), 1–18; *The Greek Theater and its Drama*⁴ (Chicago, 1936), pp. 330–7) this number will work if it comes from a chronological list of S.'s plays compiled at a time when *some* of them had been lost. (See also Pearson (1917), vol. 1, xviff.).

3. From a statement ascribed to Androtion (Jacoby 324 F 38 = *Test* 19) we learn that one of Sophocles' colleagues was Pericles. For the reason why we put S.'s generalship in 441/0 not 440/39 see Jacoby *ad loc.*

4. For date see A. Körte, *MDAI(A)* 18(1893), 246–9.

5. See M. H. Jameson, 'Sophocles and the Four Hundred', *Historia* 20 (1971), 541–68.

6. Cf. C. F. Russo, 'Euripide e i concorsi tragici lenaici', *MH* 17 (1960), 165–70, at 165–6.

7. For a bracingly sceptical approach see Mary Lefkowitz, *The Lives of the Greek Poets* (London, 1981). (See also the review of Lefkowitz by J. Fairweather (*CR* 32 (1982), 183–4), whose own article 'Fiction in the biographies of ancient writers', *AncSoc* 5 (1974), 231–75, is highly relevant.) A more traditional account of Sophocles' life is given by A. Lesky, *Die tragische Dichtung der Hellenen*³ (Göttingen, 1972), pp. 169–75.

8. Less sceptical about the historicity of the quarrel are e.g. O. Hense, *Studien zu Sophokles*

(Leipzig, 1880), pp. 289–310, and P. Mazon, 'Sophocle devant ses juges', *REA* 47(1945), 82–96.

9. For this mysterious figure see Pauly-Wissowa *RE* III.A.1. 1044–5.

10. O. Weinreich, *Antike Heilungswunder* (Giessen, 1909), pp. 38ff., sees the 'healing right hand' as the primary significance of 'Dexion', any connection with the 'welcoming' of Asclepius being secondary.

11. W. S. Ferguson, 'The Attic orgeones', *HThR* 37 (1944), 61–140, at 90.

12. U. von Wilamowitz-Moellendorff, *Der Glaube der Hellenen* (Berlin, 1931–2), vol. 2, pp. 232–3 ('dieser fromme Mann ...'); E. R. Dodds, *The Greeks and the Irrational* (Berkeley, 1951), p. 193.

13. E. J. and L. Edelstein, *Asclepius* (Baltimore, 1945), vol. 2, p. 117 n. 24; followed by H. Lloyd-Jones, *The Justice of Zeus* (Berkeley, 1971), pp. 192–3 n. 13.

14. If we insist on connecting the Asclepius story with the plays it had better be done in the cautious terms advocated by G. M. Kirkwood, *A Study of Sophoclean Drama* (Cornell, 1958), pp. 25–6.

15. There is a breathtaking example in B. Seidensticker, 'Die Stichomythie', in W. Jens, *Die Bauformen der griechischen Tragödie* (Munich, 1971), p. 209, who says in relation to *Ajax*: 'When he wrote the earliest of his surviving plays Sophocles was about 45 years old, with about twenty years' experience of the stage.' For arguments about the date of *Ajax* see App. G. to Stanford (1963), and Lesky (1972), pp. 180–1 n. 2.

16. *P. Oxy.* 2256 fr. 3, exhaustively discussed in A. F. Garvie, *Aeschylus' 'Supplices': Play and Trilogy* (Cambridge, 1969).

17. Edn of *Ajax*, lii.

18. Reinhardt (1979); the original came out in 1933 (3rd edn in 1947).

19. Cf. the review by A. Rivier (*MH* 21 (1964), 243) of E.-R. Schwinge, *Die Stellung der Trachinierinnen im Werk des Sophokles* (Göttingen, 1962). Schwinge is explicitly in Reinhardt's debt in his attempt to date *Trach.*

20. Knox (1979), pp. 112ff. For different arguments and another date (411) see C. Diano in *Dioniso* 15 (1952), 81ff.

21. On attempts to locate *Ajax* in relation to history see Johansen (1962), 171 and Winnington-Ingram (1980), p. 72 n. 38. On *Elec.* see H. Lloyd-Jones in *CR* 19 (1969), 36–8; on *Trach.* see Easterling (1982), pp. 19–23.

22. For a helpful account see App. 2 of Easterling (1982).

23. *De falsa leg.* 246.

24. (Plu.) *Vit. dec. or.* 841f.

25. Alexandria: R. Pfeiffer, *History of Classical Scholarship*, vol. 1 (Oxford, 1968), pp. 87ff. Byzantium: L. D. Reynolds and N. G. Wilson, *Scribes and Scholars* (Oxford, 1968), ch. 2; and N. G. Wilson, *Scholars of Byzantium* (London, 1983).

26. On manuscripts which preserve scholia see the *praefatio* to V. de Marco, *Scholia in Sophoclis Oedipum Coloneum* (Rome, 1952), reviewed by H. Erbse in *Gnomon* 27 (1955), 84–7; and see also R. D. Dawe, *Studies on the Text of Sophocles* (Leiden, 1973–8), vol. 1, pp. 113–19. An edn of the scholia was done by P. N. Papageorgios (Leipzig, 1888) for the Teubner series.

27. A. Turyn, *Studies in the Manuscript Tradition of the Tragedies of Sophocles* (Illinois, 1952); cf. P. E. Easterling, 'The manuscript A of Sophocles and its relation to the Moschopulean recension', *CQ* 10 (1960), 51–64.

28. Dawe (1982), p. 26.

29. Cf. his preface to *Ajax* (Leiden, 1953). K.'s subsequent reaction to Turyn – K. believes the Parisinus is not valueless – is at *Mnemosyne* 11 (1958), 25–31.

III. LANGUAGE AND STAGE ACTION

Although the career of Sophocles overlapped in its earlier years with that of Aeschylus and later on with that of Euripides, it is very hard to avoid over-simplifying the development of fifth-century tragedy into a progression *from* Aeschylus *to* Sophocles *to* Euripides. The same simplification is found amongst ancient critics, for whom Sophocles is 'the middle one' in ways which go beyond mere chronology. Thus Dio Chrysostom (first/early-second century A.D.) in his comparison of the three tragedians' versions of the Philoctetes story says of Sophocles that 'he seems to stand midway between the two others, since he has neither the ruggedness and simplicity of Aeschylus nor the precision and shrewdness and urbanity of Euripides, yet he produces a poetry that is august and majestic (σεμνὴν δέ τινα καὶ μεγαλοπρεπῆ ποίησιν), highly tragic and euphonious in its phrasing, so that there is the fullest pleasure coupled with sublimity and stateliness (μετὰ ὕψους καὶ σεμνότητος)'.[1] Approximately a century earlier the critic Dionysius of Halicarnassus also found a 'middle' quality in Sophocles' style: between the 'austere' (Pindar, Aeschylus, Thucydides, etc.) and the 'smooth' (Sappho, Euripides, Isocrates, etc.) he located the intermediate, 'well-blended' (εὔκρατος) mode of composition, including Sophocles as well as Homer, Demosthenes, Plato, and others.[2] Of this intermediate style Dionysius says he is at a loss to decide 'whether it is produced by excluding the extremes or by blending them'; but it is at any rate clear that it is defined principally by reference to what it is *not*.

The perception of Sophocles' plays as 'central', with corresponding associations of balance and harmony, is all of a piece with the frequent ancient description of him as 'sweet' and 'a honey-bee' (*Test* T IIa); already in *Frogs* (line 82) he was called εὔκολος, 'easy'. But it would be a mistake to acquiesce without more ado in the view that Sophocles' use of language constitutes a marvellous paradigm of classical 'rightness'. Before we agree that 'with a power, an ease, a skill which are the culminating achievement of the Greek genius, he employs the endless miracle of language to express and interpret, to set out in clear, faultless pattern, the fathomless miracle of life',[3] we should examine in detail some of the powerful and often disturbing effects which his language actually creates.

First: he confronts physical unpleasantness with an unflinching descriptive energy. One may mention the self-blinding of Oedipus (*Oed. Tyr.* 1276ff.), the smashing of Lichas' skull (*Trach.* 781–2), Philoctetes' suppurating wound (repeatedly in *Phil.*, but esp. 696ff., 783–4, 823–5), the stench of Polynices' corpse (*Ant.* 410–12, 1082–3), the bloody consequences of suicide by the sword (*Ajax* 917–19, *Ant.* 1238–9). But the energy is *controlled*: as Dionysius said, 'in his speeches Sophocles is not excessive (περιττός), but keeps to what is necessary (ἀναγκαῖος)'.[4]

More generally, the plays are full of startling linguistic life. Sometimes this derives from repetition. Whereas Creon told Haemon to spit Antigone out (πτύσας, *Ant.* 653) it is at Creon that he eventually spits (πτύσας, 1232): the link suggests the distance which Creon has travelled. Deianeira and Iole are both 'uprooted' (ἀνάστατοι, *Trach.* 39; ἀνάστατον, 240): the repetition draws attention to the thematically important equivalence between the situations of the two women. Sometimes the linguistic effect is due not to repetition but to the alarming appropriateness of a particular choice of word in a particular context. Thus Creon, in saying, 'Those are my general principles; in close connection with them I have made a particular proclamation about Polynices and Eteocles', uses ἀδελφός, 'brotherlike' (192), to mean 'in close connection'; and it is no coincidence that the only other comparable use of the word in Sophocles is at *Oed. Col.* 1262 – the speaker being Polynices. In *Oed. Tyr.*, words for eye recur in ways which, though they may individually seem innocent, must cumulatively, in this of all plays, strike us as unnerving (esp. 987, 1222). A further kind of impact is produced by language which 'enacts' its own meaning. Thus in *Oed. Tyr.* the contorted relationship of incest is presented in words whose syntax is itself unusual (e.g. 425, 1271–4, 1403–5),[5] and in *Trach.* the juxtaposition of words forming contrasting pairs enacts the sense of mutability which the ode is 'about'.[6] Finally one may recall even tinier cases of irrepressible linguistic life, such as the puns on the name of Haemon (*Ant.* 659, 794), the play on βίος/βιός ('life'/'bow') at *Phil.* 931 and 933,[7] and the brilliant γε at *Elec.* 1216 – the second most overwhelming use of this particle in tragedy.[8]

Much illuminating work has been done in recent decades on larger-scale aspects of Sophoclean language than the ones just discussed, especially on patterns of imagery (in the sense of recurring metaphors) running through the plays. Outstanding in this respect is Goheen's book on *Ant.*:[9] he is notably successful in showing how Antigone and Creon are differentiated by the contrasting types of image associated with each (e.g. the use by Creon of imagery from the sphere of money, merchandise, and profit – κέρδος). In *Oed. Tyr.* too imagery is an important carrier of meaning, particularly as certain images express the total reversal in Oedipus' fortunes: for example, the plague requires a doctor, which is what Oedipus claims to be (68), yet by the end of the play it is he who is revealed as the disease (1396).[10] The other tragedies have also been responsive to studies of their imagery.[11]

The danger with studies of a play's language is of course that what is actually happening, what is visible on stage, may be undervalued. In a sensible attempt to redress the balance some critics have recently been laying great emphasis on 'stagecraft' – exits and entrances, the grouping and movements of characters, the significant use of stage props, etc.[12] This approach too can be risky if pushed to extremes – it may elevate the quest for 'the original performance' into the sole critical goal, whereas the text of any play is susceptible of many realizations – yet it has much enhanced our appreciation of the tragedies.

Some of the most shattering moments in the theatre, ancient and modern, are produced by the apparently simple action of an exit or an entrance. Two notable Sophoclean exits are those of Deianeira in *Trach.*, who leaves in silence after hearing what she has done to Heracles, and Oedipus in *Oed. Col.*, whose stumbling, blind frailty changes to the certainty and calm dignity of his final, unaided departure to die. Even more overtly 'dramatic' are two memorable entrances, that of Creon carrying the body of Haemon in *Ant.*, and that of the now blind Oedipus in *Oed. Tyr.* Sometimes effects relating to entrances or exits are more complex. In *Phil.* various efforts to induce Philoctetes to leave Lemnos end in a 'frustrated' or 'false' exit; but at last, thanks to the authoritative persuasiveness of Heracles, Philoctetes acquiesces in the course of action which, though by no means unequivocally 'good', will both lead to his being healed and demonstrate a fortitude worthy of the wielder of Heracles' bow – and at this point he does make his exit.[13]

One dramatically powerful prop is Philoctetes' bow, which several times in the play allows a moral issue to become, in a literal sense, tangible; as when Philoctetes' trust is shown by his willingness to let Neoptolemus handle the bow (654ff.), or when the cruelty of the deception is made manifest in Neoptolemus' refusal to return the bow (923–6).[14] There is something comparable in *Elec.* The two most memorable scenes, namely the narrative of Orestes' supposed death and Electra's mourning of his supposed ashes in the urn, are both intensely paradoxical – superficially based on illusion, yet emotionally as genuine as anything else in the play. The culminating moment, and one which illustrates the importance of physical objects as the focus for and visual analogue of emotional or moral issues, is when Electra relinquishes the 'dead' Orestes and takes the live Orestes in her arms (1205–26).[15]

In conclusion it should be stressed that the separation of Sophocles' art into language and stage action is – of course – artificial. It is the fusion of the two from which his greatest dramatic effects derive; as in the complex deployment of the imagery of blindness and sight in the two plays which also exploit, through stage action, the contrast between the sighted and the sightless man.[16]

NOTES

1. *Or.* 52.15; tr. Crosby (Loeb).

2. *De comp. verb.* 21–4.

3. J. W. Mackail, *Lectures on Greek Poetry*[2] (London, 1911), p. 173. This is quoted by G. H. Gellie, *Sophocles: a Reading* (Melbourne, 1972), p. 261. Gellie himself discusses Sophocles' style in his ch. on 'Poetry', pp. 261–79.

4. *De imit.* 2, fr. 6.2.11 (2.206. 16–17 in Usener-Radermacher) = *Test* 120. For an author not keeping to 'what is necessary' one may compare the stomach-turning description of the self-blinding at Seneca *Oed.* 952–79.

5. There is a different effect at *Oed. Tyr.* 1184–5, where the horror of incest emerges by *contrast* with the *formality* of the Greek.

6. Cf. Easterling (1982), note on 94–140.

7. Cf. D. B. Robinson, 'Topics in Sophocles' *Philoctetes*', *CQ* 19 (1969), 34–56, at 43–4.

8. The most overwhelming is Eurip. *Bacch.* 1278.

9. R. F. Goheen, *The Imagery of Sophocles' 'Antigone': a Study of Poetic Language and Structure* (Princeton, 1951).

10. B. M. W. Knox's book *Oedipus at Thebes* (Yale, 1957) takes verbal analysis about as far as it can go (cf. the reservations of Kamerbeek at pp. 26–8 of his edition of *Oed. Tyr.*). In 'Sophocles' *Oedipus*' (in Knox (1979)) K. brilliantly but sometimes fancifully analyses the mathematical imagery in *Oed. Tyr.*, and explores the possibility that plays on the name 'Oedipus' are present.

11. See e.g. P. Biggs, 'The disease theme in Sophocles' *Ajax*, *Philoctetes* and *Trachiniae*', *CPh* 61 (1966), 223–35; D. Cohen, 'The imagery of Sophocles: a study of Ajax's suicide', *G & R* 25 (1978), 24–36 (esp. on sword imagery); W. B. Stanford, 'Light and darkness in Sophocles' *Ajax*', *GRBS* 19 (1978), 189–97; V. J. Rosivach, 'The two worlds of the *Antigone*', *ICS* 4 (1979), 16–26 (esp. on light and dark); M. G. Shields, 'Sight and blindness imagery in the *Oedipus Coloneus*', *Phoenix* 15 (1961), 63–73; P. W. Harsh, 'Implicit and explicit in the *Oedipus Tyrannus*', *AJPh* 79 (1958), 243–58; C. P. Segal, 'The hydra's nursling: image and action in the *Trachiniae*', *AC* 44 (1975), 612–17.

12. Cf. O. Taplin, *The Stagecraft of Aeschylus* (Oxford, 1977) and *Greek Tragedy in Action* (London, 1978); also W. Steidle, *Studien zum antiken Drama unter besonderer Berücksichtigung des Bühnenspiels* (Munich, 1968).

13. See Taplin (1978), pp. 67–9. On the ambiguous ending to *Phil.* see P. E. Easterling, '*Philoctetes* and modern criticism', *ICS* 3 (1978), 27–39, at 35–9.

14. Cf. Taplin (1978), pp. 89–93. Detailed analysis of stage action in *Phil.* can be found in Taplin, 'Significant actions in Sophocles' *Philoctetes*', *GRBS* 12 (1971), 25–44.

15. It is noteworthy that we cannot say for sure precisely when Electra does let go the urn. Jebb (followed by D. Seale, *Vision and Stagecraft in Sophocles* (London, 1982), p. 71) thinks it happens between 1217 and 1218 – and this would be one possibility for a director to consider. The passage is in any case a useful reminder that the stage action is *not* always entirely deducible from the words.

For more on the urn scene see J. Dingel, 'Requisit und szenisches Bild in der griechischen Tragödie', in Jens (1971), pp. 355ff.

16. Cf. R. G. A. Buxton, 'Blindness and limits: Sophokles and the logic of myth', *JHS* 100 (1980), 22–37, and Seale (1982). (Note in passing the importance of touching in the plays: e.g. *Oed. Tyr.* 1510, *Oed. Col.* 1638–9.)

IV. HEROES IN THE DRAMA: THE PROBLEM OF 'CHARACTER'

The idea that what happens on stage in a Sophoclean play should be interpreted above all in the light of the motives and intentions of the individual characters has had and continues to have widespread support. In the words of one critic who adopted such a character-oriented approach, 'Sophocles differs from the other two tragedians in directing his whole technique to the presentation of one or at most two great figures'.[1] But in recent years the notion of 'character' has come under increasingly critical scrutiny. In this chapter we shall examine some of the issues involved.

Anyone who reads Sophocles with even a cursory attentiveness is bound to notice that several of the plays share a common pattern, according to which a major dramatic figure displays heroic but often ruthless fixity of purpose, refusing to heed the dissuasions of those around him or her. The intransigence of Ajax, the relentless pursuit of truth by Oedipus (in *Oed. Tyr.*), the single-mindedness of Antigone (in *Ant.*) and of Electra, the stubbornness of Oedipus (in *Oed. Col.*) – these qualities all may be seen as exemplifying 'the heroic temper'.[2] One may single out the rousing uncompromisingness of *Ajax* 479–80, *Ant.* 96–7 (contrast the non-heroic 'common man' at *Ant.* 439–40) and *Elec.* 986–9; in *Trach.* Deianeira, in spite of beginning the play as a passive victim, achieves a kind of heroism later (n.b. 721–2); in *Phil.* Sophocles returns time and again to the question of what it is to possess a heroic φύσις (nature);[3] and it is clear that the issue was not confined to the extant plays (frr. 87 and 808 Radt). But it is a big step to go from this to the conclusion that Sophoclean dramas centre on a 'hero', in the sense in which one might say that the hero of *Hamlet* is Hamlet. Or if one does take the step, difficulties present themselves. Who is the 'hero(ine)' of *Trach.*? If Antigone is the 'heroine' of *Ant.*, why does she disappear from dramatic interest towards the end as the action centres on Creon? If Ajax is the 'hero' of *Ajax*, what do we make of the last third of the play when he is already dead? And who on earth is the 'hero' of *Phil.*?

In fact few questions are less interesting than 'Who is the hero of ... ?' This is clear enough in relation to *Phil.*, that intricate ballet of interrelationships. But there might seem to be more excuse for asking it about *Ant.* and *Trach.*, and for feeling some puzzlement about *Ajax*. Faced with the shifts of emphasis in these plays, some critics have adopted the term 'diptych'.[4] But this does no more than redescribe the very thing which needs explaining. More productive is the approach advocated by John Jones.[5] Taking his cue from Aristotle's statement in *Poetics* that tragedy is the 'imitation of an action', πράξεως ... μίμησις (1449b 36–7, cf. 1450a 16–17), Jones discussed a number of Greek plays and showed how much more sense they make if we accord primacy not to 'character' but to 'action'. This insight revealed as illusory some of the problems which had been bothering Sophoclean scholars. Thus *Ant.* portrays neither 'the things done and suffered by Antigone' nor 'the things done and suffered by Creon', but an action: the events unleashed by Creon's proclamation. Again, *Trach.* centres neither on Deianeira nor on Heracles but on an action: the sequence of events leading to the downfall of Heracles. Even *Ajax*, which may arguably be read as 'the things done and suffered by Ajax', yields a more complete response if we recognize as its subject the sequence of events which unfolds as a result of Ajax's attempt on the lives of his commanders – for that sequence reaches its conclusion not with Ajax's death but with the granting to him of burial.[6]

Not only did Jones wish to reduce the interpretative importance of character in favour of action: he also, more radically, doubted whether one ought to ascribe to figures on the Greek stage a personality with a 'self-maintained continuity'[7] of the sort exhibited by, say, Macbeth. One good reason for entertaining such doubts is the masking convention of Greek drama.[8] When we realize that Antigone and Electra (like all the female characters) were played by men; that Heracles and Deianeira were most likely played by the same actor; and that the part of Theseus in *Oed. Col.* would have been played in turn by two or even three actors,[9] then we are forced to abandon the continuity which we often (even after Brecht) assume between actor and role, and to recognize that a 'character' is something constructed by a dramatist, not a person with an independent existence. We have thus learned to think twice before giving a psychological answer to a question of the type, 'Why does such-and-such a character say such-and-such?' An example is the question, 'Why does Ajax, in the "deception speech", say that he will give way?' The assumption behind this is that Ajax's words should be interpreted in the light of his motives and intentions which his words enable us to reconstruct. But it may be that a more sensible question is, 'Why does Sophocles have Ajax make this speech?'[10] Or again, we might wish to substitute for the question, 'Why does Oedipus blind himself?' the alternative, 'Why does Sophocles present Oedipus as blinding himself?'[11]

Various attempts have been made to 'dissolve' character, by making it a function of other elements in the drama. One by no means novel procedure is to see consistency of character as something subordinate, liable to be sacrificed to the 'effectiveness' of particular scenes;[12] the danger here is that concentrating on local dramatic effects may lead one to undervalue what a play is actually about and to reduce drama to melodrama. Another approach, and a subtle and valuable one, urges us to see 'character' as shaped by the dramatic form of a play. Much work has been done, especially by scholars writing in German, on the formal structure of Greek tragedy, including description of such apparently isolable features as prologue, *parodos*, choral *stasima*, *stichomythia*, *rhesis*, and *amoibaion*.[13] Less common has been application of such formal analysis to the interpretation of the plays. A now famous Euripidean instance of this type of approach is Miss Dale's discussion of the twofold dying-scene in *Alcestis*: the 'same' experience is explored through lyric song and then in spoken iambic trimeters, the contrast being a matter not of 'change of mind' but of a switch in dramatic perspective, like the alternation between recitative and aria in opera.[14] Comparable shifts in formal perspective occur in Sophocles.[15] In *Ajax*, sung expressions of grief during an *amoibaion* are followed by an ordered (but still passionate) *rhesis* at 430ff.; in *Elec.* the heroine's feelings are explored successively in monody, *amoibaion*, and *rhesis* (86–309); in *Ant.* Antigone's reaction to her imminent death is presented first through *amoibaion* and then in *rhesis* (806–928).

An important contribution to the debate on dramatic form has been made by J. Gould. He notes Sophocles' tendency to 'run over' formal distinctions – in contrast to Euripides, who tends to emphasize the separateness of *rhesis*, prologue, etc. – the result being that we are 'enticed into seeing dramatic action as unfolding process and development, one phase growing from another, and personality is correspondingly experienced as in some degree continuous and developing'.[16] Thus, even when we take account of the various modes in which individual personalities are presented, we seem to be led back once more to the impression of a continuity in Sophoclean characters; and – in the case of Sophocles at least – the gap between 'dramatic formalists' on one side, and champions of 'humanly intelligible' and psychologically comprehensible characters on the other, may conceivably be bridgeable.[17] However, there is no point in denying that a vigorous disagreement is taking place here, a disagreement which is not due to the narrowness or obtuseness of the critics concerned, but which reflects the complexity of the issues under discussion. There is no scholarly consensus, and the outcome of the argument is uncertain. Just for that reason, the problem of 'character' is one of the most fascinating to confront the student of Sophocles at present.

NOTES

1. T. B. L. Webster, *An Introduction to Sophocles*[2] (London, 1969), p. 55.

2. I borrow the phrase from B. M. W. Knox's perceptive and sophisticated book *The Heroic Temper: Studies in Sophoclean Tragedy* (Berkeley, 1964).

3. E.g. 79ff., 88–9, 94–5, 874–5, 902–3, 971, 1013–15, 1310ff., 1371–2. The general question of φύσις in Sophocles is the starting-point of H. Diller's essay 'Über das Selbstbewusstsein der sophokleischen Personen', *WS* 69 (1956), 70–85 (repr. in Diller's *Kleine Schriften zur antiken Literatur* (Munich, 1971), pp. 272–85.

4. Cf. A. J. A. Waldock, *Sophocles the Dramatist* (Cambridge, 1951), pp. 49ff., following Webster (1969), p. 102, etc. Diptychs threaten to invade even the satyr-plays, too fragmentary to defend themselves: cf. D. F. Sutton, *The Greek Satyr-Play* (Meisenheim, 1980), pp. 45 and 47.

5. *On Aristotle and Greek Tragedy* (London, 1962).

6. Reinhardt (1979), pp. 30 and 36, has some excellent remarks on what binds *Ajax* and *Trach.* into dramatic wholes. On *Ajax* see also A. C. Pearson, 'Sophocles, *Ajax*, 961–973', *CQ* 16 (1922), 124–36; J. Tyler, 'Sophocles' *Ajax* and Sophoclean plot construction', *AJPh* 95 (1974), 24–42; Segal (1981), p. 432 n. 5.

7. Jones (1962), p. 37.

8. See Sir A. Pickard-Cambridge, *The Dramatic Festivals of Athens*[2], revised by J. Gould and D. M. Lewis (Oxford, 1968), index *s.v.* 'masks'. The whole book is an invaluable guide to details of staging, actors, costume, audience, etc.

9. See Pickard-Cambridge (1968), pp. 142–4.

10. For one answer see Charles Garton, 'Characterisation in Greek tragedy', *JHS* 77 (1957), 247–54, at 252.

11. For a possible answer see Buxton (1980); also ch. 4 of A. Cameron, *The Identity of Oedipus the King* (New York, 1968).

12. The classic proponent of this view is Tycho Wilamowitz, *Die dramatische Technik des Sophokles* (Berlin, 1917). For a discussion of Tycho see H. Lloyd-Jones in *CQ* 22 (1972), 214–28.

13. See Jens (1971); important reservations about the isolability of the components are to be found in Taplin (1977), esp. pp. 49–60 and 470–6.

14. See Eurip. *Alc.* ed. A. M. Dale (Oxford, 1954), note on 280ff.; also introduction, pp. xxii–xxix. For the comparison with opera see J. Gould, 'Dramatic character and "human intelligibility" in Greek tragedy', *PCPhS* 204 (1978), 43–67, at 50–1, and M. Black, *Poetic Drama as Mirror of the Will* (London, 1977).

15. See B. Mannsperger, 'Die Rhesis', in Jens (1971), pp. 173–4.

16. Gould (1978), 51. One may compare B. Seidensticker, 'Die Stichomythie', in Jens (1971), p. 206: commenting on the difference between Aeschylean and Sophoclean stichomythia, he notes that Sophocles mixes kinds of stichomythia which are distinct in Aeschylus.

17. See P. E. Easterling, 'Presentation of character in Aeschylus', *G & R* 20 (1973), 3–19 (followed by Winnington-Ingram (1980), 6–8), and 'Character in Sophocles', *G & R* 24 (1977), 121–9; also Garton (1957).

V. MEANING

(a) *Gods and humans*

When we describe a work as 'tragic', one of the things we may imply is that in it human conduct is presented in counterpoint with forces beyond mankind's control. In Greek tragedy this metaphysical dimension[1] is supplied not by fate (a concept pretty well irrelevant to Greek tragedy)[2] but by the purposes and actions of the gods. To a greater or lesser extent all Sophocles' plays incorporate these purposes and actions as part of the drama. However, although there is general agreement that divine-human relations constitute an area crucial for our understanding of Sophocles, critics differ widely over how to interpret those relations.

It will be convenient to start from the case argued by Bowra. His opinion was that 'the central idea of a Sophoclean tragedy is that through suffering a man learns to be modest before the gods.'[3] The religious content of the plays thus becomes unequivocally didactic: 'Sophocles allows no doubts, no criticism of the gods . . . If divine ways seem wrong, human ignorance is to blame. In the end the gods will be proved right'.[4] Perhaps because it corresponds to the traditional notion of Sophocles as a pious old gentleman, Bowra's interpretation has proved remarkably tenacious. Yet it is open to grave objections. First, it drastically underestimates the weight accorded by Sophocles to the heroic striving of mortals for their ideals and against all obstacles.[5] Sophocles in fact spends far less time on the attitudes of the gods than on those of the humans. Of course the picture varies from play to play: at one extreme is *Elec.*, where the actions of the gods have virtually no part in the drama;[6] at the other is *Ajax*, where Athene herself appears at the outset. But even in *Ajax* Athene recedes. What is important is how the mortals react to Ajax; it is through mortals that some kind of resolution is finally achieved.

Secondly, the pietist approach makes the gods' involvement seem far clearer than it really is. The purposes of the Sophoclean gods are usually enigmatic, Athene in *Ajax* and Heracles at the end of *Phil.* being the only exceptions. For the rest, when the divine will does become an issue it is normally available only through fallible human intermediaries. What matters is how humans *perceive* the gods' intentions; as in the case of the oracle in *Phil.*, which 'varies' in accordance with the way it is apprehended and used by humans (see ch. VII, p. 32). In *Ant.* there is little doubt that what Antigone is doing is in accordance with the requirements of ritual, but there is certainly doubt about whether the gods are felt to take any part in assisting in the burial (cf. 278–9, 421). About the gods' attitude to Oedipus in *Oed. Tyr.* we have no evidence – that is not what the play is about.[7] The situation is similar in *Oed. Col.*: the voice which summons Oedipus to his death is strange and awesome, but to read into it notions of final blessing, grace, etc. is wholly unwarranted (see ch. VII, p. 30). In *Trach.* the relationship of the gods' purposes to the action is again obscure, and the work offers a particularly complex exploration of how things happen. Among those to whom responsibility for events may legitimately be ascribed are Heracles, Deianeira, Nessus, and Kypris/ Aphrodite (cf. 441ff., 488–9, 497ff., 860–1); yet the last line affirms that 'There is none of these things that is not Zeus'.[8] This is plainly not intended to *replace* the ascriptions of motive throughout the play, but it reminds the audience that the most enigmatic presence of all behind the action is Zeus himself. His power and authority are un-questioned (436–7, 1022, 1086ff., 1185, 1188), and the chorus at the beginning of the play feels confidence in his concern for mortals, or at least for his own children (139–40). But by the end the mood has changed: Heracles draws attention to Zeus' distance ('Zeus amid the stars', 1106) and Hyllus reflects bitterly on the gods' apparent lack of concern (1264ff.). The enigma remains: it is impossible to be sure what tone to read into 'There is none of these things that is not Zeus', whether one of accusation or, more likely, of a sad realization that 'that's the way the world is'. But to read it, with the pietists, as 'whatever is, is right' fails to do justice to the disturbing complexity of Sophocles' vision.

(b) *Irony and limits: making sense of the pattern*

Irony has traditionally, and rightly, been regarded as one of Sophocles' hallmarks. It is not just a technique; it is at the very heart of his per-ception of experience. Irony of tone and irony of situation have in com-mon a gap between the apparent and the real.[9] In an ironical remark the speaker is aware of and exploits the gap; in an ironical situation he or she is (often blithely) unaware of it. Irony is thus a powerful tool for a dramatist who wishes to explore the gap between partial and full knowledge and to examine the limits of human insight. In other hands than Sophocles', irony might create a sense of cosy superiority shared by author and audience/readers vis-à-vis the characters; with Sophocles, the audience is typically in the far from cosy situation of a horrified, spell-bound, and helpless crowd watching someone walk unknowingly towards a precipice.

Oed. Tyr. teems with unnerving moments of irony, perhaps the most crushing of all being at 1178, where the shepherd says that he saved baby Oedipus out of pity. Until the revelation of the truth Oedipus' ignorance is cast into ironical relief by the blind but insightful Teiresias; when the truth comes out the irony instantly dissipates, to be replaced by the horror of full knowledge.[10] In *Ajax* irony is used to emphasize man's limited vision when in the first scene the power and superiority of Athene is contrasted with Ajax's self-confident unawareness. *Elec.* too deploys irony, not only in the scene where Aegisthus is deceived about the identity of the corpse, but more centrally during the episodes when Electra is led to believe in Orestes' death through the narrative of the chariot-race and the scene with the urn.[11] Since Deianeira, Hyllus, and Heracles all at different points make grievous misjudgements on the basis of inadequate knowledge, there is much scope for irony in *Trach.* The most memorable instance is Deianeira's singling out of Iole for pity, in ignorance of who she is (307ff.); the most eerie is the dying centaur's advice to Deianeira: 'Once you have used the charm on Heracles, he will never look at another woman and love her more than you' (576–7). *Ant.* does not rely to the same extent on irony, though the downfall of Creon certainly involves the related ideas of 'learning too late' (see below) and limitation of vision. In *Phil.* too irony plays a fairly minor role. It is certainly at work in the poignant scenes where Philoctetes bestows his trust on the deceitful Neoptolemus, but in general *Phil.* is not a play in which the audience looks on from a vantage-point of knowledge: the audience (as was suggested earlier) is deliberately kept in doubt about the requirements of the oracle and is several times surprised by the turn of events on stage. Nor is irony prominent in *Oed. Col.*: very early on Oedipus knows not merely as much as the audience but more than they.

   While the extent to which irony is deployed varies from play to play, a perception closely related to the ironic perspective – the perception that human life is fragile and limited – is fundamental to his dramas. Nowhere (excepting in *Oed. Tyr.* – cf. 1186–1222, esp. 1189–92)[12] is this sense of limitation more forcefully present than in *Ajax*. Not only is there Ajax's humiliation before Athene at the outset; we also have the quieter insights afforded by the morally authoritative Odysseus, who near the beginning likens mortal life to a shadow (125–6) and near the end affirms that what we all have in common is a grave (1365). Usually – for this is tragedy – the perception of limit comes ὀψέ, too late. This is cruelly true for Deianeira: she acts misguidedly, realizes too late, and kills herself. (Heracles also recognizes too late what the pattern is, but his case is less morally interesting.)[13] In *Oed. Tyr.* first Jocasta and then Oedipus realize, horribly late, how the past fits together. In *Ajax* and *Ant.* late-learning is linked to another Sophoclean motif, the feeling that events are at a crisis; the precariousness is conveyed through the metaphor of the razor's edge (*Ajax*

786; *Ant.* 996).[14] The temporal urgency is externally contrived in *Ajax* thanks to the arbitrary restriction of Athene's anger to one day; but in *Ant.* the fact that Creon comes 'too late' to save Haemon and Antigone is integral to his character. He has shown limited vision throughout; he *would* come too late.[15]

If we add the sense of limit to the relentless and unbowed figures characteristic of the Sophoclean stage, the mixture takes us a long way towards appreciating the particular quality of this dramatist. But one further element should be noticed: 'mutability'.[16] It is expressed at the end of the parodos of *Trach.*, when the chorus sings of the ceaseless alternation of πῆμα and χαρά, woe and joy, which Zeus has ordained for mortals (126ff.) A related perception is prominent in *Ajax*, where we see an enemy who turns into a friend (Odysseus), and hear how nothing is stable and all things give way, one to another (646ff.). This rhythm at the heart of things finds dramatic expression in a famous Sophoclean ploy, the juxtaposition of scenes of rejoicing with those of sadness or horror (e.g. *Ajax* 693ff., *Oed. Tyr.* 1086ff., *Trach.* 205ff., and cf. *Ant.* 1115ff.).[17] The violent emotional effects produced by such contrasts are not meretricious, precisely because they mirror the meaning: the plays are *about* the alternations of human fortune, the dramatic structure *enacts* that alternation.[18] The notion of an alternating rhythm is echoed in a subsidiary theme, that of 'the dead killing the living', as with Hector's sword in Ajax[19] and the murder of Heracles by Nessus in *Trach.*[20] This rhythm of action and reaction is not a matter of right and wrong. What happens to, say, Haemon is not *just*. But then, if it were, this would not be tragedy.

(c) *Politics*

Attempts to detect in Sophocles' plays allusions to contemporary political events have on the whole turned out to be unconvincing.[21] But politics in its etymological sense – how one should behave in a *polis*; what living in, or being deprived of, a *polis* means – these issues are present and often prominent. Indeed the fullest recent study of Sophocles[22] takes as its theme the way in which the plays explore the contrast between civilization (exemplified by the *polis*) and the wildness within which civilization is set, and which forms a boundary or threat to it. But as usual we must be careful not to flatten out the differences between plays; we shall look at each work in turn.

In *Ant.* the *polis* is central. For Creon – so he would have us believe – the good of the *polis* is the supreme good (cf. his admirable-sounding inauguration speech, 162–91). Yet is the *polis* simply coextensive with its ruler's will? After all, the edict forbidding Polynices' burial is a proclamation by Creon, not a law passed by the

Theban assembly (e.g. 8, 27, 32, 34, 192, 447, 450, 453–4). And surely Creon's emphasis on obedience in the city (e.g. 666–7, 734ff.) goes too far? One of man's achievements may be the temperament which permits him to dwell in cities (355–6), but such communities generate the tragic tensions examined in *Ant.*

A contrast found in *Ant.* (370) is that between the person who is ὑψίπολις, 'high-citied', and the one who is ἄπολις, without or apart from a city. *Oed. Col.* examines this latter state. Oedipus has no *polis*. The helplessness of his situation emphasizes the inexpressible value of belonging to a community; it also acts as a commentary on the Thebans, who ejected him, and on Theseus, who accepts him as a fellow-citizen of Athens. Although *Oed. Col.* does not raise particular questions about the institutional running of a state (contrast Eurip. *Supp.*) it does deal with general matters of political behaviour as embodied in the distinctions between persuasion, trickery, and violence.[23]

Ajax is not set in a *polis*, but it is about the relation of an individual to a community. According to one interpretation the central character is seen as

unfit for the new age, the political institutions which impose rotation and cession of power, which recognize and encourage change ... Ajax belongs to a world which for Sophocles and his audience has passed away – an aristocratic, heroic, half-mythic world which had its limitations but also its greatness ...[24]

On that reading *Ajax* becomes deeply representative of Greek tragedy as a whole, which is a retelling in the fifth-century Athenian *polis* of events from the mythical world of heroes.[25]

Phil. too is about an individual and a community; as in *Ajax*, that community is the Greek army at Troy. The central tension in the play is between Philoctetes' desire to rejoin human society and his bitterness at having been cast out from it. Even more than in *Oed. Col.*, the contrasting moral-political implications of persuasion, deception, and violence are prominent dramatic issues.[26]

In *Elec.* and *Trach.* the main focus of attention is on the household rather than the *polis*, but in *Oed. Tyr.* the two contexts are fused, since Oedipus is king as well as husband and father. The public aspect of his downfall gives it added significance: the reversal is that much more 'exemplary' (cf. 1193–6) as the depth of the fall is greater. But *Oed. Tyr.* is not centrally *about* politics.[27]

NOTES

1. Cf. A. Rivier, *Essai sur le tragique d'Euripide*[2] (Paris, 1975), pp. 140–1.
2. The relevance of the concept of fate to Greek tragedy has been urged by Thomas Gould in an article on *Oed. Tyr.* (*Arion* 5 (1966), 478–525) and in Gould (1970). His arguments are

stimulating, but he tends to lump together 'fate' and 'the gods', obscuring the fact that, while the latter recur constantly in Greek tragedy, the former very definitely does not.

3. C. M. Bowra, *Sophoclean Tragedy* (Oxford, 1944), p. 365.

4. Bowra (1944), p. 367.

5. C. H. Whitman, *Sophocles: a Study of Heroic Humanism* (Cambridge, Mass., 1951) represents the opposite pole to Bowra; cf. Johansen (1962), 152ff.

6. Cf. Segal (1981), p. 290.

7. See E. R. Dodds' outstanding article, 'On misunderstanding the *Oedipus Rex*', *G & R* 13 (1966), 37–49, repr. in his *The Ancient Concept of Progress* (Oxford, 1973), pp. 64–77. The idea that the gods *deliberately humiliate* Oedipus has been shown to be quite untenable: cf. the criticisms of Bowra (1944) in Waldock (1951), pp. 149ff.

8. On the speaker – most probably the chorus – see Easterling (1982), ad loc.

9. See D. C. Muecke, *The Compass of Irony* (London, 1969) and *Irony* (London, 1970).

10. On sight/blindness/irony see Buxton (1980), Seale (1982).

11. On deception in Sophocles see U. Parlavantza-Friedrich, *Täuschungsszenen in den Tragödien des Sophokles* (Berlin, 1969).

12. See R. W. B. Burton, *The Chorus in Sophocles' Tragedies* (Oxford, 1980), pp. 178–9.

13. Cf. introduction to Easterling (1982), p. 6.

14. Cf. *Elec.* 22; *Oed. Col.* 88–95, 1508; *Trach.* 82, 164ff., 173–4. For the importance of 'the moment of crisis, the *kairos* or *akme*' in *Elec.* see T. W. Woodard, '*Electra* by Sophocles: the dialectical design (Part II)', *HSPh* 70 (1965), 195–233, at 201.

15. The contrast between *Ajax* and *Ant.* is made brilliantly by Reinhardt (1979), p. 91.

16. I borrow the word from Jones (1962); see his index for references.

17. On *Oed. Tyr.* see D. Sansone, 'The third stasimon of the *Oedipus Tyrannos*', *CPh* 70 (1975), 110–117; on *Ant.*, see Burton (1980), pp. 132–4.

18. Contrast Puccini in Act IV of *La Bohème*, where the sad dénouement is preceded by some high jinks, the sole rationale of which is to serve as a foil for what follows.

19. The sword was a counter-gift for the belt given by Ajax to Hector – itself an instrument of death. See Jebb's excellent note on *Ajax* 1031.

20. *Trach.* 1159–63. For the theme see H. D. F. Kitto, *Form and Meaning in Drama* (London, 1956), pp. 193–5. Note also frr. 210. 24ff. and 211. 10ff. (Radt): the spear of Achilles healed Telephus; Telephus in return promised that he and his kin would not help the Trojans; but Telephus' son broke the promise; so the son of the dead Achilles kills the son of Telephus with Achilles' spear. Did Sophocles use the motif of 'the dead getting revenge'?

21. On this type of approach see Johansen (1962), 163–4. Some examples: R. G. Tanner, 'The composition of the *Oedipus Coloneus*', in *For Service to Classical Studies: Essays in Honour of Francis Letters*, ed. M. Kelly (Melbourne, 1966), pp. 153–92; C. Diano, 'Sfondo sociale e politico della tragedia greca antica', *Dioniso* 43 (1969), 119–30 (most of this volume records a congress on social-political aspects of the ancient theatre); W. M. Calder, 'Sophoclean apologia: *Philoctetes*', *GRBS* 12 (1971), 153–74. The best-known reading of Sophocles with one eye on fifth-century history is V. Ehrenberg, *Sophocles and Pericles* (Oxford, 1954).

22. Segal (1981).

23. See R. G. A. Buxton, *Persuasion in Greek Tragedy: a Study of 'Peitho'* (Cambridge, 1982), pp. 132–45.

24. Knox (1979), 148.

25. The doubleness of tragedy is a central theme of J.-P. Vernant and P. Vidal-Naquet, *Tragedy and Myth in Ancient Greece* (Eng. tr. Brighton, 1981).

26. Cf. A. F. Garvie, 'Deceit, violence and persuasion in the *Philoctetes*', in *Studi classici in onore di Quintino Cataudella* (Catania, 1972), vol. 1, pp. 213–26; Buxton (1982), pp. 118–32.

27. A different view is taken by Knox (1979), p. 93, where it is argued that Oedipus represents Athens, 'the city which aimed to become (and was already on the road to becoming) the *tyrannos* of Greece …'

VI. THE CHORUS

(a) *The chorus and the action*

Though lacking the pre-eminence which it apparently had earlier in the development of tragic drama,[1] the chorus remained a central element in the plays of Sophocles.[2] We find in his works, as in those of Aeschylus and Euripides, that counterpoint between heroes and chorus which is a major aspect of the doubleness of Greek tragedy.[3] The fates of Oedipus, Ajax, Heracles, and the rest are not private or claustrophobic (contrast Seneca); on the contrary, they are played out in public, before groups of ordinary people. These groups, again as in the other tragedians, are socially or politically marginal: women (*Elec.*, *Trach.*), old men (*Ant.*, *Oed. Col.*, *Oed. Tyr.*), subordinates (*Ajax*, *Phil.*). The identity of the groups, far from being a matter of indifference, may materially affect the way in which the plot of the drama is inflected. We know from Dio Chrysostom (*Or.* 52.15) that, whereas Sophocles' chorus comprised sailors who had come along with Odysseus and Neoptolemus, Aeschylus and Euripides brought on a chorus of inhabitants of Lemnos. It can hardly be doubted that in choosing as he did Sophocles intended to emphasize Philoctetes' utter isolation.

Unlike the heroes, the chorus neither experiences tragic dilemmas nor takes tragic decisions. Its business is not to choose (cf. *Ajax* 165–6, *Oed. Col.* 294–5, *Phil.* 1072–3), rather to react and to reflect. But we should beware of regarding these reflections as reflective – as cool or uninvolved. It has been well pointed out, for instance, that the Sophoclean chorus characteristically arrives on stage in a mood of uncertainty or agitated questioning: Is the rumour true? (*Ajax*) Why are you still crying? (*Elec.*) What has become of the intruder? (*Oed. Col.*) What has Apollo said? (*Oed. Tyr.*) What can I say, how help? (*Phil.*) Where is Heracles? (*Trach.*)[4] Moreover, as the action unfolds the choral response to it may be very intense: ἔφριξ' ἔρωτι, περιχαρὴς δ' ἀνεπτάμαν, 'I shudder with passion, I take wing for joy,' sing Ajax's men on hearing what they take to be a sign of their leader's change of heart (693). Even when a chorus does rise above the particularity of the action to draw out its more general significance, the language used frequently indicates a passionate involvement with that particularity: ἰὼ γενεαί βροτῶν ... ὦ τλᾶμον Οἰδιπόδα ... ὦ Ζεῦ ... ἰὼ κλεινὸν Οἰδίπου κάρα ... τάλας ... ἰὼ Λάϊειον ⟨ὦ⟩ τέκνον ..., 'Alas the generations of mortals ... O miserable Oedipus ... O Zeus ... Alas, famous Oedipus ... wretched one ... Alas, O child of Laius ...' (*Oed. Tyr.* 1186ff.).

The Sophoclean chorus does not, then, stand emotionally aloof from the action. But it does on several occasions offer a wider, even a profounder perspective from which the context and meaning of the stage events may be more fully appreciated. Two good examples are in *Trach*. In the *parodos* (94–140) we receive a sustained impression of the alternation which is manifest both in natural phenomena and in human fortunes, and we confront the question of how Zeus' purposes relate to human life in general and to Heracles' life in particular. Then at 497–530 we meet three memorable images: invincible Kypris, with her umpire's staff of authority; Heracles, locked as usual in a combat with monstrosity; and Deianeira, the passive spectator who is like a deserted calf. These two choral songs allow us to see beyond the mortal agents by offering us a glimpse of the forces to which those mortals are subject.

But (in extant Sophocles) the choruses too are mortal; and their vision, like that of the heroes, is limited.[5] So when they react and reflect it is by no means always from a vantage-point of superior insight – witness the soldiers' misplaced joy at Ajax's supposed relenting (*Ajax* 693ff.) or the Thebans' optimistic but soon-to-be-crushed speculations about Oedipus' parentage (*Oed. Tyr.* 1086ff.). Nor, more interestingly, is it always the case that the chorus' attitude is 'ideal' in relation to the audience's evaluation of the moral action. At a local level this applies to some of the stylized two-line punctuation marks by which the chorus respectfully and impartially notes the end of major speeches, perhaps to urge prudence (*Elec.* 990–1, 1015–16) or to caution against excessive rancour (*Ajax* 1091–2, 1118–19).[6] But it applies also to more pervasive aspects of the attitudes of certain choruses, for instance the horror of the old men in *Oed. Col.* when they learn the identity of the stranger (e.g. 226, 233–6) – a horror which is cast into relief by the nobler reaction of Theseus (551ff.). The chorus must not be assumed to be 'the mouthpiece of Sophocles' – *all* the words of *all* the stage figures were written by him. Even when choruses set their seal on a play with a concluding generalization, this must never be assumed without more ado to be the play's 'message'; it is just one piece of the total picture.[7]

It is from the complex interrelation of individual heroes and collective chorus that the drama derives. Obviously that interrelation differs from play to play, and to generalize about a 'typical' choral attitude in Sophocles is to court disaster. But it may be helpful to cite the remarkable words which Reinhardt uses to illuminate the relationship of the chorus to Antigone's lament (*Ant.* 801ff). He describes the short choral passages interspersed through her song as 'not echoing, not reinforcing, but standing out in contrast – a kind of frame, or like two banks on either side, between which the lament runs like a stream, or like groups of people standing on the bank and following with their eyes someone who is being snatched away by the current. That is how the chorus stands in safety and watches, participating, but outside'.[8] One may quibble – what is sweeping Antigone away is not an impersonal current but something which is, at least in part, a product of human wills. Yet Reinhardt's image brilliantly conveys the role played by the chorus in so many Greek tragedies, that of a deeply-concerned *observer* of suffering.

(b) *Form*

It is a truism that we miss a good deal of the effect of Greek tragedy through not having the original music or choreography. Nevertheless we can to some extent compensate for this if we attend to the formal, especially metrical, richness of the plays. The handling of the chorus is a major factor in the creation of this richness. Now what strikes one about Sophocles in this respect – and it is surely, on its own, enough to silence anyone who believes Greek tragedy was a ritual (in the sense of a ceremonial repetition of a fixed pattern) – is the tremendous formal variety which we find, even in so small a sample as seven works.

As an instance of this variety we may take the *parodos* and what immediately follows it. In *Ajax*, after an iambic prologue which itself exhibits great formal flexibility so far as the length of the speeches is concerned, we have a sequence of choral anapaests, followed by a lyric triad (strophe/antistrophe/epode). Then comes an interchange between Tecmessa and the chorus (201ff.): she keeps to anapaests, while they switch from anapaests to sung lyrics when they hear what has happened to Ajax (221ff.). In *Ant.* the *parodos* consists of lyric sections interspersed with anapaestic sections; it is followed by a scene in iambics. *Oed. Tyr.* and *Trach.* each have their *parodos* in sung lyrics, but even here there is diversity: *Oed. Tyr.* has three pairs of strophe/antistrophe, *Trach.* has two such pairs, plus an epode. The pattern in *Elec.* is different again. An anapaestic solo by Electra leads into a sequence of three lyric strophe/antistrophe pairs, with a concluding epode. Within this framework there is a combination of antiphonal regularity and subtle diversity: the strophes, the antistrophes and the epode all begin with the chorus and end with Electra, but the division between singers occurs at a different point in each of the pairs and in the epode. It is important to realize that in this scene in *Elec.* we are not confronted with metre for metre's sake: the metre binds Electra and the chorus together – contrast *Ajax* 348ff., where Ajax's lyrics are sharply distinguished from the calmer iambic voices of the chorus and Tecmessa. In the *parodos* of *Phil.* we find something analogous with the *Ajax* scene just mentioned, since (yet another pattern) there is a contrast between the agitated lyrics of the sailors and the calmer anapaests of Neoptolemus. Finally there is the amazing *parodos* of *Oed. Col.* Although its structure is not outwardly difficult to grasp (two strophic pairs; epode; song by Antigone) that structure accommodates an extraordinary range of emotion and, above all, movement, both literal and metaphorical. At the end of a long artistic career Sophocles' technical mastery was at its height.

It would not be hard to work through the plays illustrating at length how in Sophoclean choral utterances form is used for expressive effect. In the space available we can do no more than mention a few representative examples. One such occurs towards the end of *Ant.* At 1261–76 and 1284–1300 Creon sings a lyric lament as he carries his son's body in his arms. Each part of the lament has in its midst a single line of choral comment, in iambics. The more everyday mode of utterance offsets the anguish of the song.[9] A comparable effect is created at *Oed. Tyr.* 1313ff., where the blinded Oedipus utters a combination of dochmiacs and iambics, while the chorus remains wedded to iambics. (Compare *Elec.* 1232–87: Electra's excitement at the recognition is enacted in lyric, while Orestes' greater restraint shows itself in iambics – at least until 1280, when he shares a line of lyric *antilabe*.) On formal aspects of the chorus in *Phil.* the main point to make is a large-scale one, namely that there is in the play only one extended choral song (676–729). That this should be so is entirely fitting: since the chorus is closely implicated in the intrigue, it would be inappropriate for it constantly to be standing back from the action and reflecting upon it. Lastly we may note another passage in *Oed. Col.* Although 1447–99 is less complex than the scene at 117ff., it is still a good example of form controlled in the service of meaning. On the face of it the structure is one of almost mathematical regularity: strophe; five iambic trimeters for actors; antistrophe; five trimeters; strophe; five trimeters; antistrophe. Moreover the sets of trimeters are themselves exactly parallel: two lines for Oedipus; one for Antigone; two for Oedipus. But within this order there are subtle variations. In the second strophic pair the proportion of dochmiacs to sung iambics is greater than in the first pair, matching the chorus' increased excitement; and the point within strophe/antistrophe at which the thunder-claps are registered is different each time.[10]

In general, what is notable about Sophocles' use of choral speech and song is his flexibility, and his prodigality of invention. As with so many of the conventions of Greek tragedy, the metrical forms should be seen not as restricting what can be said, but as the very conditions which allow dramatic statements to be made.[11]

NOTES

1. 'Apparently': because the early history of tragedy, hazy at the best of times, became hazier still with the downward revision of the dating of Aeschylus' *Suppliants* (cf. ch. II n. 16 above). (A sensible discussion of the origins of tragedy is now available in the *Cambridge History of Classical Literature*, vol. 1 (Greek), 258ff.) 'Pre-*Suppliants*' but still essential as a study of the development of the chorus is W. Kranz, *Stasimon* (Berlin, 1933); also useful, on this as on other matters relating to the chorus, is Pickard-Cambridge (1968), ch. 5.

2. Cf. G. M. Kirkwood, 'The dramatic role of the chorus in Sophocles', *Phoenix* 8 (1954), 1–22.

3. Cf. ch. V n. 25 above.

4. See J.-U. Schmidt, *Sophokles: Philoktet. Eine Struckturanalyse* (Heidelberg, 1973), pp. 57–8.

5. On the tricky matter of the 'limitations' of the chorus see H. Lloyd-Jones' review of G. Müller's commentary on *Ant.*, *CR* 19 (1969), 25. There has been a good deal of controversy, in relation to *Ant.*, about how far the chorus' views are 'in character' and how far they go beyond it: cf. G. Müller, 'Überlegungen zum Chor der Antigone', *Hermes* 89 (1961), 398–422; B. Alexanderson, 'Die Stellung des Chors in der Antigone', *Eranos* 64 (1966), 85–105; P. E. Easterling, 'The second stasimon of *Antigone*', in *Dionysiaca*, ed. R. D. Dawe, J. Diggle and P. E. Easterling (Cambridge, 1978), pp. 141–58.

6. On this convention of even-handedness see Burton (1980), p. 35.

7. Sophocles' liking for a choral *diminuendo* at the end of a play is discussed by D. A. Hester, 'Very much the safest plan, or last words in Sophocles', *Antichthon* 7 (1973), 8–13.

8. Reinhardt (1979), p. 82.

9. See Burton (1980), p. 135.

10. See Burton (1980), p. 269.

11. For help with the details of tragic metre one may with profit turn to A. M. Dale, *The Lyric Metres of Greek Drama*² (Cambridge, 1968) and M. L. West, *Greek Metre* (Oxford, 1982).

VII. PARTICULAR INTERPRETATIVE PROBLEMS

In what follows I shall look either at competing interpretations of an entire play, or at a more specific issue or issues – whichever seems the more useful in a given case. The works are ordered alphabetically.

Ajax

Sometimes a problem arouses so much interest that the criticism relating to it becomes self-perpetuating. This has happened with the 'deception speech' (646–92), now the object of a minor industry.[1] But in spite of the conflicting advice one can make some progress.

A good place to begin is the preceding scene. By the end of it it is plain that, as far as Tecmessa is concerned, Ajax is resolved to die. He has said goodbye to his son, giving him his shield – 'the other armour will be buried along with me' (577). He tells the women not to cry in his presence: such a dirge is inappropriate where what is called for is the knife (581–2). Tecmessa begs him to relent, but he refuses (591–5). 'He would be better dead,' sings the chorus (635), and that outcome is surely now expected. Instead we have 646–92: 'Everything changes, and so shall I. I will obey the Atreidai; I will soften.' The chorus is joyfully convinced that Ajax has changed his mind (715–18). Then we learn that his fate is in the balance (786); Athene's anger pursues him for one day only – he must not be left alone (796). But alone he is, thanks to a dramatic device rare in tragedy, namely the removal of the chorus. He announces that he has *not* relented, and commits suicide. Now it is clear that the *effect* of 646–92 is to deceive Tecmessa and the chorus about Ajax's plans. But was that also his intention? The question has been much debated, because many critics wish to rescue Ajax from the imputation of 'lying'. Yet it is not clear to the present writer why this is thought to matter so much: no one in this play makes 'always telling the literal truth' the measure of the hero; it is small beer besides trying to murder one's superiors.

As usual, more rewarding than the question, 'Why does Ajax make this speech?' is, 'Why does Sophocles give Ajax this speech?' This brings us to change. Are we to read Ajax's generalizations about it as applying to himself? If so, the message is, 'As the whole world is subject to the law of change, so must I be'; if not, the message is, 'All the world is subject to the law of change, but I am not.' The latter view is argued eloquently by Reinhardt;[2] the former is put most subtly by Sicherl, who argues that, paradoxically, Ajax's death *is* his withdrawal, his act of submission, his acceptance of change.[3] The issue is complex, but the likelihood is that Reinhardt's account is preferable:

Ajax's dying curse (835ff.) and Teucer's refusal to let Odysseus touch the corpse (1393–5) give a strong sense of the *persistence* of Ajax's wrath. Moreover, the motifs of 'only for one day' and 'do not let him alone' are instructive. It is as if *given time* Ajax could be retrieved from his isolation. But his death intervenes; there has not (for this is a tragedy) been time for him to bend.

Antigone

It seems agreed that the main critical issue is: how do we evaluate the respective moral positions of Antigone and Creon. Provided this is not asked in order to achieve 'that nice apportionment of blame to which critics are so much more prone than dramatists',[4] but rather with the aim of teasing out just what is at stake between the two principal figures, the question is worthwhile.

Defenders of Creon appear from time to time.[5] There is no doubt that some of the sentiments he expresses, particularly in his opening programmatic speech, are laudable in themselves (e.g. 182–3); nor should there be any doubt that Creon receives some measure of sympathy as he carries his son's body on stage at the end. But is his original proclamation (it is not a law – cf. ch. V(c) above) morally acceptable? Teiresias' dire warnings strongly suggest it is not. There has been much argument about how Creon's edict related to Athenian law,[6] but certain points are clear: although there was apparently nothing abnormal in the denial of burial in his homeland to a traitor (cf. e.g. Thuc. 1. 138; Plu. *Mor.* 834a), not only was there a custom, specifically associated with Athens, according to which one should not pass a corpse by without placing some dust upon it (Aelian *V.H.* 5. 14; *N.A.* 2. 42; Cic. *De leg.* 2. 25. 63),[7] but also, in forbidding Polynices burial *anywhere*, in actively ensuring that his body be torn apart by dogs and birds, Creon plainly went too far.

Most critics accept the moral impropriety of Creon's proclamation and disagree only in the degree (or absence) of qualification which they allow in their approval of Antigone. For some the approval is absolute;[8] others, believing grey to be a more interesting colour than black and white, stress problematic aspects of her behaviour – harshness towards Ismene, relentless concern with honour, etc.[9] A beneficial corollary of the latter approach is that, by emphasizing the particularity of Antigone's character, it makes us less likely to reduce the play to an opposition between principles – city *versus* kin-bond, state *versus* individual, or whatever. Neither Creon nor Antigone is the vehicle for a simple idea: 'the theme of ... *Antigone* ... [is] the tragedy of two human downfalls, separate in nature, ... following one another as contrasting patterns.'[10]

Electra

Elec. poses none of the problems about dramatic unity which bother some critics of *Ajax*, *Ant.*, and *Trach.* If any play is unified through its main character, this one is. The interpretative difficulties mostly concern not form but morality. *Elec.* portrays the events leading up to two murders, one a matricide. The plan apparently has divine approval (32ff.), and its eventual success is celebrated by the chorus as an achievement of freedom (1508–10); and there the action ends. What do we make of a work which seems to present in so unproblematical a light the killing of a mother?

One way round this is to deny the premise, i.e. to assert that the matricide *is* problematic. A recent advocate of this course, noting a number of allusions to the Furies, and assuming that 'the pursuit of Orestes was an established part of the legend',[11] presents a case for our seeing what happens on stage as the working out of 'Fury-justice', a process which there is no reason to think must end where the play does. Again, study of the play's imagery has suggested a progression from light to darkness;[12] and a corresponding development has been detected in the moral action, from an assumption that the plotted vengeance is just (32ff.) to a situation where the reality turns out to be very different.[13] It has even been doubted whether we are to make that initial assumption of Apollo's support for Orestes: reservations range from the moderate ('nowhere in the play does Apollo give explicit and unambiguous sanction for the matricide')[14] to the extreme (Orestes' question to the oracle is 'impiously' dishonest)[15]. Now it is true that on emerging after the murder of Clytemnestra Orestes once expresses doubt about the rightness of Apollo's advice (1424–5).[16] But thereafter, instead of dwelling remorsefully on the deed, Orestes is involved in more action; and the harshness of Aegisthus, for instance his language of cruelty and enforcement (1461–3), strengthen our sympathies for Orestes and Electra. It would seem that *Elec.* is a play in which the significance of the ending may legitimately be moulded by a director in either a positive or negative sense without his being false to the text. (One may compare the differently ambivalent endings of *Phil.* and *Trach.*) It is worth adding that, if the positive inflection is adopted,[17] the seriousness of the work as a whole is not thereby undercut. Thanks to the portrayal of Electra, *Elec.* remains 'a drama of suffering, powerlessness, cruelty, noble immoderation, both in hate and love'.[18]

Oedipus at Colonus

One central theme of *Oed. Col.* links it to the earlier works: an isolated figure demonstrates unswerving fixity of purpose in the face

of adversity. One aspect of this theme, namely the confrontation between a community-less individual and a community, closely recalls
Phil., and in a different way *Ajax*. Also shared with *Phil.*[19]
are the importance of 'locality';[20] the feeling that the hero is, in spite
of his resilience, potentially responsive to loving counsel (that of
Neoptolemus and Antigone); and the dramatic exploration of persuasion, violence, and cunning as contrasting types of moral action.[21]

Two specific issues in the critical debate may be raised here. First,
the end: is Oedipus' passing to be seen as in some sense a reconciliation
with the gods? Second, the progress to the end: is the play
'episodic', and, if so, do the episodes merely 'delay' the attainment
of the play's climax?

As for the end, one critic speaks of 'a sublime reconciliation not
merely between Oedipus and the gods but between all the warring
elements in the situation',[22] while another discerns the presence of
'divine grace' and 'redemption'.[23] If this is correct, it means that the
enigmatic Sophoclean gods have at last become clearer, their relation
to human justice being at last made manifest. But care is needed.
Oedipus is not going up to 'heaven', he is going to Hades (1547–8,
1551–2, 1554–5, 1556ff.). True, the chorus prays that, after all his suffer-
ings, Oedipus may be exalted again by a 'just *daimon*' (1565–7), but –
leaving aside the point that this is a prayer and not a statement of fact
– the chorus has no doubt that Oedipus will *die* ('Let him go down
to the land of the dead without harassment from Cerberus', 1568ff.).
His passing is not triumphant, but mysterious: we are unsure whether
his death was accomplished thanks to the mediation of the gods above
or those below (cf. 1654–5, with Jebb's fine note; 1661–2), but that
he has died is certain (1689ff., 1701, 1706, etc.). For *Oed. Col.* as for
other dramas Sophocles wrote an ending which is far too finely balanced
to be called happy or sad.[24]

A forthright proponent of the 'episodic' view wrote thus: 'The story
of Oedipus' death did not contain stuff for a play ... there was this
superb climax in sight, but not much to lead up to the climax'. So
Sophocles had to find something suitable for 'filling out the middle
of the play'.[25] Such an approach fails to do justice to *Oed. Col.* It is
a play about a man's gradual progress from utter isolation to a state
of being accepted. It charts the crossing of a series of boundaries: from
sacred grove to lawful ground, from outside a *polis* to inside it, from
life to death. It surrounds this progress with contrasting moral and
political alternatives: Athens or Thebes? Deceit or persuasion? Reject
Polynices unheard, or yield to Antigone and hear him out? It is through
such choices (and those faced by Theseus) that the significance of the
climax is built up. Only after watching the long and emotionally

anguished course travelled by Oedipus can we appreciate the impact of his decision willingly to die in the territory of Athens.[26]

Oedipus Tyrannus

Of all the plays, this is the one which has elicited the most widely discrepant interpretations. It has been argued that Oedipus must have known the truth all along;[27] on this it is enough to refer to the conclusive counter-arguments of B. Vickers.[28] It has been argued that Oedipus was a helpless puppet without any free will; this view has been undermined by E. R. Dodds, who reminds us that *Oed. Tyr.* portrays a man choosing his course of action.[29] It has been argued that *Oed. Tyr.* is based on a set of coincidences so fantastic in their improbability that 'we should as reasonably fear to be hit by a thunderbolt as to be embroiled in his particular set of misfortunes';[30] but it is essential to remember that the moral which the chorus draws from Oedipus' fate is not, 'How astonishing a run of bad luck', but, 'Taking your *daimon* as an example, Oedipus, I call no mortal happy' (1193–5) – that is, Oedipus' fate *typifies* man's fragility. (One may compare Kafka's eerie story *Die Verwandlung* ('Metamorphosis'), in which a man wakes to find that he has turned into a giant louse. It is even less likely that one of Kafka's readers should become a giant louse than that one of Sophocles' audience should suffer the misfortunes of Oedipus; yet in both cases the artist makes worthwhile the leap of imagination by the reader/spectator.) Then there are those who, following Freud, see merit in applying the 'Oedipus Complex' to *Oed. Tyr.*;[31] against this we may cite the delightfully persuasive paper by J.-P. Vernant,[32] who points out the crucial fact that, until disabused by the Corinthian (1016ff.), Oedipus believes his parents to be Polybus and Merope – so he can hardly have had a Complex about Laius and Jocasta. Lastly we may mention the view according to which the entire plot hinges on a false detail planted by Sophocles – the story, to which Oedipus clings, that Laius was killed by several men.[33] But – if necessary – eloquent psychological justification can be provided for the detail ('Is it contrary to human nature for a man to cling with all his intelligence to a hope, however faint, and argue desperately on the strength of it?');[34] and it may be suggested that in any case uncertainty over number, like uncertainty over the oracles in *Phil.*, is merely a particular example of mankind's generally inadequate knowledge.

Philoctetes

This is the most dramatically intricate of the plays. Sometimes this intricacy has been interpreted as improvisation on the part of the playwright,[35] but it is better to follow the trend of recent criticism and

regard the false starts and changes of direction in *Phil.* not as the results
of hasty composition but as integral to the play's meaning. *Phil.*
presents mortals acting on the basis of imperfect and piecemeal
knowledge, trying to make reasonable guesses about the future.[36] The
audience too, apart from having a general notion of the outcome, is
uncertain about how things will develop. This is relevant to the question
of the oracle, on which several scholars have recently concentrated.
One view used to be: the oracle prescribed the use of persuasion; this
was ignored by Odysseus; hence his plan failed.[37] But no one in the
drama makes this point,[38] and anyway the audience is not sure what
the oracle's precise provisions are.[39] Oracles are a mode of contact with
the gods, but so heavily do they rely on the interpretations of human
intermediaries that they illustrate (or are used by Sophocles to illustrate)
the shakiness of human knowledge.

Another point of debate is how we take the final part of *Phil.*, when
Philoctetes is on the verge of leaving to return home to Greece but
is then persuaded by Heracles to go to Troy. From one angle it is the
departure for Greece which is the 'right' ending. Neoptolemus begins
by using deception but 'grows up' to honesty and the use of persuasion;[40] as a result, trust is re-established between him and Philoctetes; thus for Neoptolemus now to be persuaded by Philoctetes is
a fitting tribute to the reciprocity of their new relationship.[41] A further
reason for regarding departure for Greece as a poetically just conclusion is the harsh treatment which Philoctetes has suffered at the
hands of the Greek army, exemplified by Odysseus' behaviour within
the play. But, on the other hand, we want Philoctetes and Neoptolemus
to go to Troy, where healing and glory await. The ending is, in other
words, balanced between hope and sadness.[42] Given the extreme suffering to which Philoctetes had been exposed, it could hardly be other-
wise.

Trachiniae

In 1959 a leading expert on Greek tragedy wrote that *Trach.* 'is
usually the least esteemed, though not the least enjoyed, of the plays
of Sophocles'.[43] Today that lack of esteem no longer applies. We seem
now to be more receptive to the violent emotions which lurk beneath
and sometimes burst out from this work. Scholars aware of develop-
ments in anthropology have alerted us to the uneasy tension between
the barbarous and the civilized, the wild outside and the sheltered inside, which runs through *Trach.*;[44] and growing scepticism about
Sophoclean piety has enabled us to respond with more accuracy to
the play's bleak dramatic landscape.

The most interesting problems of interpretation concern the ending.

If we see Hyllus' marriage to Iole as a restitution of order after chaos and as a healing of the house of Heracles, and if we take Heracles' fate to be not death in agony but apotheosis in glory, then the tone of the play's final moments will seem to be relatively harmonious. If we dwell on the insensitivity of Heracles' instructions, and emphasize not the brief allusions to Mt. Oeta but the prospect of Heracles' anguished death, then we have an altogether more bitter conclusion.

Take the apotheosis first. Excavations on Mt. Oeta have revealed offerings to Heracles from the archaic to the Roman periods, together with a square area with a layer of ash 40-80cm. deep.[45] Presumably then the allusion to Heracles' pyre in *Trach.* would have been accepted by the audience as matching the known reality of a cult. We know too from literature and art that the story of the apotheosis was in circulation before Sophocles' time.[46] What we do not know for certain is whether, when *Trach.* was put on, there was already a story that Heracles achieved divinity through the pyre.[47] But, even if there was, we have no right to allow such a version to flood in and drown the details as Sophocles himself wrote them.[48] The fact is that he could have made Heracles' end unambiguously glorious, but he did not. As with the conclusions of other plays (*Phil., O.C.*), the tone is ambivalent between hope and despair.[49]

'Brutal' is an epithet which many would apply to Heracles' command that Hyllus marry Iole.[50] Much emphasis is laid by Sophocles on Hyllus' reluctance, a fact which cannot be disguised even if we recognize that the audience 'knew' Hyllus and Iole to be the ancestors of the illustrious Heraclidae. So what are we to make of Hyllus' reaction? What he says is that Iole alone is responsible for the death of Deianeira and the downfall of Heracles.[51] Well, the play has indeed shown that love – love for Iole – was one cause of the tragedy. But there are other causes: the characters of Deianeira and Heracles, the resentment of Nessus, not to mention (possibly) Zeus. So, although we feel with Hyllus, we cannot fully share his judgement of Iole; nor, therefore, can we fully share his horror at Heracles' order. To that extent, one element of the work's concluding bitterness is mitigated.

Postscript

My decision to conclude this booklet with a chapter in which each play is dealt with separately was a deliberate one, since in the last analysis it is with individual works that appreciation is concerned. But this format, together with the unavoidable brevity of my comments, has drawbacks. I am well aware that my approach might be taken to imply that 'the problems' are isolable and finite, and that in order to solve them one has simply to choose between the alternatives which critics have already put forward. In fact, of course, 'the problems' alter as scholarship itself develops, and my account of the state of play is necessarily a provisional one. It is certain that in thirty years' time those who think about Sophocles will be asking different questions from those we ourselves are disposed to ask. It is impossible to predict whether those questions will be generated by new movements in literary studies, in anthropology, in history, or in some quite different branch of enquiry. But that so powerful a genius as Sophocles will indeed be a focus for continuing discussion is beyond doubt.

Thanks to the best recent scholarship, the tenacious image of a 'genial, serene, dignified graybeard' has been undermined, to be replaced by something altogether more unsettling. If only the validity of this reappraisal might be more often tested in the place where Sophocles belongs: the theatre.

NOTES

1. Segal (1981), pp. 432–3 n. 9 gives an idea of the bibliography.

2. Reinhardt (1979), p. 24; cf. also 'The *Ajax* of Sophocles' in Knox (1979).

3. M. Sicherl, 'The tragic issue in Sophocles' *Ajax*', *YCS* 25 (1977), 67–98; for a variant of this see Taplin (1978), pp. 127ff.

4. Winnington-Ingram (1980), p. 75.

5. E.g. W. M. Calder, 'Sophokles' political tragedy, *Antigone*', *GRBS* 9 (1968), 389–407.

6. See D. A. Hester, 'Sophocles the unphilosophical', *Mnemosyne* 24 (1971), 11–59, for large bibliography; also H. Petersmann, 'Mythos und Gestaltung in Sophokles' Antigone', *WS* 91 (1978), 67–96. On refusal of burial in Greece see now Jan Bremmer, *The Early Greek Concept of the Soul* (Princeton, 1983), pp. 90ff.

7. Cf. Petersmann (1978), 92–3.

8. Müller (1967), p. 11: 'Antigone hat ganz und gar recht, Kreon hat ganz und gar unrecht'; on this see Knox (1979), p. 166.

9. For some references see Segal (1981), p. 444 n. 50. How far the *chorus* is critical of Antigone is a moot point, the resolution of which is bound up with a detailed linguistic argument (e.g. about 853–6). A. Lesky does not think they are critical of her (*Gesammelte Schriften* (Bern, 1966), pp. 176–84); Burton (1980), p. 125 disagrees.

10. Reinhardt (1979), p. 65. For *Ant.* as comprising two interdependent and equally important downfalls see J. C. Hogan, 'The protagonists of the *Antigone*', *Arethusa* 5 (1972), 93–100.

11. Winnington-Ingram (1980), p. 226.

12. See in particular C. P. Segal, 'The *Electra* of Sophocles', *TAPhA* 97 (1966), 473–545.

13. Seale (1982), p. 79. According to H. F. Johansen, the play 'ends, as it began, in a distressing atmosphere of uncertainty' ('Die Elektra des Sophokles', *C & M* 25 (1964), 8–32, at 29).

14. Segal (1981), p. 280.

15. J. T. Sheppard, '*Electra*: a defence of Sophocles', *CR* 41 (1927), 2–9, at p. 4. Sheppard's view finds a supporter in Kells (1973), pp. 4 ff.; but it is still surely untenable. Nobody in the play suggests that Orestes should have asked 'Ought I to kill my mother?' The lines about

the oracle are about as unemphatic as they could be. (When Sophocles wants to, he is perfectly capable of making an address to Apollo memorable, cf. 637ff., 1376ff.)

16. On the degree of doubt see Kamerbeek ad loc.

17. As recommended recently by P. T. Stevens, 'Sophocles: *Electra*, doom or triumph?' *G & R* 25 (1978), 111–20.

18. Reinhardt (1979), p. 135.

19. Similarities between *Oed. Col.* and *Phil.* are noted by L. Campbell, *Sophocles*[2] (Oxford, 1879), vol. 1, pp. 260ff.

20. Cf. the chapter on *Oed. Col.* in Jones (1962).

21. Cf. ch. V n. 23 above.

22. Bowra (1944), p. 355.

23. A. Lesky, *Greek Tragedy*[2] (Eng. tr. London, 1967), p. 129.

24. For a non-triumphant reading see I. M. Linforth, 'Religion and drama in *Oedipus at Colonus*', *Univ. of Cal. Publ. in Class. Philol.* 14.4 (1951), 75–191, at 180–4.

25. Waldock (1951), p. 219. The inadequacies of the 'filling out' approach are well high-lighted by P. Burian, 'Suppliant and saviour: Oedipus at Colonus', *Phoenix* 28 (1974), 408–29.

26. On the very end of *Oed. Col.* see also Burton (1980), p. 272, where stress is laid on the sense of loss conveyed by the concluding lamentations.

27. Cf. P. Vellacott, *Sophocles and Oedipus* (London, 1971).

28. *Towards Greek Tragedy* (London, 1973), pp. 496ff. A. Lesky, in *AAHG* 20 (1967), 208, is briefer (with reference to an earlier paper by Vellacott): 'Damit ist natürlich das Kunstwerk verfehlt'.

29. Dodds (1966). See also ch. V n. 2 above.

30. Waldock (1951), pp. 159–60.

31. E.g. D. Anzieu, 'Oedipe avant le complexe', *Les Temps Modernes* 22 (1966), no. 245, 675–715. This reading is a comprehensively psychoanalytical one. ('In order to make sense of the drama of Oedipus it is necessary to assume an incestuous relationship between Creon and Jocasta, and jealousy on the part of Oedipus towards his wife's and his mother's brother' – p. 695.)

32. 'Oedipus without the Complex', in Vernant and Vidal-Naquet (1981), pp. 63–86.

33. The discrepancy between 'one' and 'many' is highlighted by Wilamowitz-Moellendorff (1917), pp. 79–80.

34. Reinhardt (1979), pp. 119–20.

35. Waldock (1951) entitles his chapter on the play 'Sophocles improvises'.

36. Cf. Robinson (1969), 47.

37. Bowra (1944), p. 265; K. Alt, 'Schicksal und φύσις im Philoktet des Sophokles', *Hermes* 89 (1961), 141–74, at 143.

38. Cf. Waldock (1951), pp. 200ff. See also Steidle (1968), pp. 169–70; Buxton (1982), pp. 129–30.

39. Easterling (1978), 27.

40. For *Phil.* as an exploration of Neoptolemus' growth to social adulthood see Vidal-Naquet's article on the play in Vernant and Vidal-Naquet (1981). That Neoptolemus does not grow *psychologically* is argued by H. Erbse, 'Neoptolemos und Philoktet bei Sophokles', *Hermes* 94 (1966), 177–201.

41. Cf. Steidle (1968), p. 190.

42. See Easterling (1978), 36–7.

43. D. W. Lucas, *The Greek Tragic Poets*[2] (London, 1959), p. 145. The wording at this point is the same as in the 1st edn (1950), p. 130.

44. See especially C. P. Segal, 'Sophocles' *Trachiniae*: myth, poetry, and heroic values', *YCS* 25 (1977), 99–158.

45. *BCH* 44 (1920), 392; cf. M. Nilsson, 'Der Flammentod des Herakles auf dem Oite', *ARW* 21 (1922), 310–16, repr. in his *Opuscula Selecta* (Lund, 1951–60), vol. 1, pp. 348–54.

46. P. E. Easterling, 'The end of the *Trachiniae*', *ICS* 6.1 (1981), 56–74, at 65–6.

47. Cf. Easterling (1981), 66.

48. Compare M. Ewans, *Wagner and Aeschylus* (London, 1982), p. 56, who makes some excellent comments on the audience's 'provisional knowledge' of the stories dramatized in Greek tragedy.

49. More on the apotheosis in Segal (1977), 138ff. and (1981), pp. 99–100.

50. The word is used by Seale (1982), p. 208; he softens it in his n. 47. On the startling idea that Heracles here shows his *love* for Iole (Bowra (1944), pp. 142–3) see the criticism of J. K. MacKinnon, 'Heracles' intention in his second request of Hyllus: *Trach.* 1216–51', *CQ* 21 (1971), 33–41, at 33–4.

51. Note that no squeamishness is expressed about son and father uniting with the same woman: the sexual issue does not arise. Incidentally, the situation is paralleled mythically when Odysseus' son Telegonus marries Penelope, and Telemachus marries Circe; cf. Apollodorus, ed. Frazer (Loeb) vol. ii, fn. on p. 303, and vol. i, p. 269 with fn. 4; also Radt (1977), p. 375, on *ΟΔΥΣΣΕΥΣ ΑΚΑΝΘΟΠΛΗΞ*.

BIBLIOGRAPHICAL KEY: BOOKS AND ARTICLES CITED MORE THAN ONCE

BOWRA (1944): C. M. Bowra, *Sophoclean Tragedy* (Oxford).

BURTON (1980): R. W. B. Burton, *The Chorus in Sophocles' Tragedies* (Oxford).

BUXTON (1980): R. G. A. Buxton, 'Blindness and limits: Sophokles and the logic of myth', *JHS* 100, 22–37.

BUXTON (1982): R. G. A. Buxton, *Persuasion in Greek Tragedy: a Study of 'Peitho'* (Cambridge).

DAWE (1982): R. D. Dawe, edn of *Oed. Tyr.* (Cambridge).

DODDS (1966): E. R. Dodds, 'On misunderstanding the *Oedipus Rex*', *G&R* 13, 37–49; repr. in his *The Ancient Concept of Progress* (Oxford, 1973), pp. 64–77.

EASTERLING (1978): P. E. Easterling, '*Philoctetes* and modern criticism', *ICS* 3, 27–39.

EASTERLING (1981): P. E. Easterling, 'The end of the *Trachiniae*', *ICS* 6.1, 56–74.

EASTERLING (1982): P. E. Easterling, edn of *Trach.* (Cambridge).

GARTON (1957): C. Garton, 'Characterisation in Greek tragedy', *JHS* 77, 247–54.

GOULD (1978): J. Gould, 'Dramatic character and "human intelligibility" in Greek tragedy', *PCPhS* 204, 43–67.

GOULD (1970): T. Gould, translation (with commentary) of *Oed. Tyr.* (Englewood Cliffs).

JENS (1971): W. Jens, *Die Bauformen der griechischen Tragödie* (Munich).

JOHANSEN (1962): H. F. Johansen, 'Sophocles 1939–1959', *Lustrum* 7, 94–288.

JONES (1962): J. Jones, *On Aristotle and Greek Tragedy* (London).

KELLS (1973): J. H. Kells, edn of *Elec.* (Cambridge).

KNOX (1979): B. M. W. Knox, *Word and Action* (Baltimore).

LESKY (1972): A. Lesky, *Die tragische Dichtung der Hellenen*³ (Göttingen).

MÜLLER (1967): G. Müller, commentary on *Ant.* (Heidelberg).

PEARSON (1917): A. C. Pearson, *The Fragments of Sophocles* (Cambridge).

PETERSMANN (1978): H. Petersmann, 'Mythos und Gestaltung in Sophokles' Antigone', *WS* 91, 67–96.

PICKARD-CAMBRIDGE (1968): Sir A. Pickard-Cambridge, *The Dramatic Festivals of Athens*², revised by J. Gould and D. M. Lewis (Oxford).

RADT (1977): S. Radt, *Tragicorum Graecorum Fragmenta*, vol. 4, *Sophocles* (Göttingen).

REINHARDT (1979): K. Reinhardt, *Sophocles*, Eng. tr. (Oxford).

ROBINSON (1969): D. B. Robinson, 'Topics in Sophocles' *Philoctetes*', *CQ* 19, 34–56.

SEALE (1982): D. Seale, *Vision and Stagecraft in Sophocles* (London).

SEGAL (1977): C. P. Segal, 'Sophocles' *Trachiniae*: myth, poetry, and heroic values', *YCS* 25, 99–158.

SEGAL (1981): C. P. Segal, *Tragedy and Civilization: an Interpretation of Sophocles* (Harvard).

STANFORD (1963): W. B. Stanford, edn of *Ajax* (London).

STEIDLE (1968): W. Steidle, *Studien zum antiken Drama unter besonderer Berücksichtigung des Bühnenspiels* (Munich).

TAPLIN (1977): O. Taplin, *The Stagecraft of Aeschylus* (Oxford).

TAPLIN (1978): O. Taplin, *Greek Tragedy in Action* (London).

VERNANT and VIDAL-NAQUET (1981): J.-P. Vernant and P. Vidal-Naquet, *Tragedy and Myth in Ancient Greece*, Eng. tr. (Brighton).

WALDOCK (1951): A. J. A. Waldock, *Sophocles the Dramatist* (Cambridge).

WEBSTER (1969): T. B. L. Webster, *An Introduction to Sophocles*² (London).

WILAMOWITZ-MOELLENDORFF (1917): T. von Wilamowitz-Moellendorff, *Die dramatische Technik des Sophokles* (Berlin).

WINNINGTON-INGRAM (1980): R. P. Winnington-Ingram, *Sophocles: an Interpretation* (Cambridge).